I0504233

PROSTATE CANCER

Living your best life

By David Dale

This book is dedicated to the men have lost the battle against prostate cancer, and the men like myself who have been victorious.

David Dale

Each day is the beginning of a new life, to live and be better than yesterday.

JAMES ALLEN

CHAPTER 1

The Doctors Appointment

This was a routine doctors appointment like many others before. Sparky, (Jordan Sparks), a new intern, what I call her was looking at my medical records with a puzzled look on her face. Then she spoke about a PSA test not being in my records. She asked if I ever had one done. I could not remember specifically having a PSA blood work done. She said she would like to order the test for me because of my age. Sure I replied, your drawing blood from me anyway why not. Blood was drawn a few days later. At my next visit I was told my numbers were elevated. With a reading of 5.6 and that she was going to send me to a urologist, which she recommended one. I made the appointment and discussed what could be the possible reasons for the elevated numbers. Mona (urologist) decided to order another PSA test to confirm there was no mistakes made in the first test. I scheduled a follow up appointment to discuss the results. I was very nervous on my way to the appointment at the possibility of having cancer.

I sat patiently for my name to be called. After I was called I was taken into small room and my vitals checked including blood pressure. The nurse assistant told my pressure was high. I looked at her sarcastically as if to say well I am here to receive possibly the worse news I ever received in all my life.

The assistant left the room and said the doctor will be with you in a minute and stepped out of the room. That minute turned into what seemed like hours. It was taking longer than usual, which lead me to believe it was a positive test result. My heart was beating pretty hard now just wanting to get it over good or bad. The door opened and the doctor entered. She gave me the bad news and I was relieved a little just to know the results. She explained my options after explaining my Gleason score and where the cancer appeared to be in the prostate gland. Then ordered more test to be done MRI's, and CAT scans of the area. A good attitude is required to tolerate some of the testing. For example lying on a table for forty-five minutes without moving is a challenge when they are injecting dye in you that you can feel.

However medical science has changed a bit for the better. The same test use to be done with a probe in your rectum. That is being phased out. It still done at certain hospitals and testing facilities. Make sure you find one with the updated technique. The testing is to make sure there is no cancer present in any other parts of your body.

I had those test done and scheduled another meeting to discuss the results with the doctor. My wife was present to hear my options.

Then Mona, went over the details of my case and recommended the I have it removed. However there were other options. One would be radiation treatments with what is called seeds. Wherein radiation pellets are inserted in the prostate gland to keep the cancer from growing or progressing. It also requires you to come into the office from time to time to get reseeded. I didn't like the idea of radiation being in my body everyday at all.

I requested more information and she set up and appointment with a radiologist group at Christiana Hospital to discuss my situation in more details. We waited in a little room for over an hour for the doctors to come in. I was already nervous and that made me even more nervous. Three people enter the room with me and my wife. Two doctors and a person taking notes. After they went over the details of my particular situation I was left with two options radiation treatments or a robotic prostectomy (removal of the prostate by robotics). I asked the two young doctors each, what would they do if they were in my situation. Both paused and said they didn't know. That made me angry inside because you guys look at these cases everyday and you don't have a clue. To me it should have been easier for them to make a decision than. So either they didn't want to answer for professional reasons or they were not good doctors. In any case they asked me to go with them to another room. I followed them to he room where they wanted to examine my prostate with there finger. I was asked to assume the position and I declined to cooperate. I already know I have prostate cancer, I have already had every imaging study (x-ray) possible to show the condition of my prostate. Why would I let you stick your finger up my ass again, for what purpose. Just so you can bill me for it and add it to your resume list of examinations performed. They lost there professional demeanor and smirked a little when I declined. As I was leaving the room the two stayed as if to have a conversation I looked back and they were smiling and talking to each other. Which let me know I was right about them. They were young fool doctors not really concerned about me. I was just a number to them, a formality to get there experience.

CHAPTER 2

The Nerves

The conversation about nerves should be discussed in detail with your surgeon if you do have prostate cancer. Whether or not they can be spared is important. The prostate gland has nerves attached to it. The nerves provide the capability for a man to achieve erections. The testing will reveal if cancer has spread to the nerves. You have two bundles of nerves attached to the Prostate gland. If cancer is present in the nerves they will have to be removed along with the prostate gland. Of course everyones condition is different depending on the extent of the cancer. The doctors first priority is to remove all cancer to save your life, lowering the risk of a reoccurrence and then nerve sparing. Although its not all or nothing, sometimes they only have to take one bundle or a portion of a bundle. Thats another important reason to know as soon as possible. The longer you wait, your not only flirting with your life but potentially, your quality of life after surgery. The other thing is all doctors don't see the same things in the X-rays, CAT scans or MRI's. Meaning one doctor may look at the results and say, I see cancer here and there. Surgeons with more, or less experienced may see the test results differently based on there experience level.

In any case I would go with most experienced doctor you can find with a good record. Hopefully you know a few folks who have had the surgery, and are satisfied with the result. The first Urologist I contacted has performed this surgery 400 times which I thought more than qualified her. My second opinion had performed the operation 4,500 times and rated one of the top ten in the United States, and his father was a surgeon in the urology field also. And he was talking less evasive surgery than the first doctor to boot. Also known as saving the nerve bundles, and my quality of life. My wife and I both liked that idea. The moral to the story is always get a second opinion when its major surgery if you have time, period.

CHAPTER 3

Surgery Day

At first I wasn't going to attend the pre operation class to discuss with, and hear from gentlemen who have had the surgery and there experiences with the whole process, but I was glad after I did. Plenty of valuable information was imparted to my wife and I about what to expect before and after surgery during our session. There is a bowel prep which is a laxative to clean you out to make surgery go easier for the doctor. No eating after six o clock the day before surgery and even that last meal should be lite since you will be taking a laxative right after that. Similar to a colonoscopy preparation.

My dad called to wish me well and to tell me not to worry everything will be ok. He wanted to come to but he is 85 years old and on dialysis three times a week. I wouldn't want him up there waiting around all day sleeping in chairs anyway.

Surgery day started early at least for me, I was up at 6:00 am for the 10:00 am appointment. I removed my wedding ring and necklace and put them in the jewelry box. My wife was stirring as she heard me moving around getting ready. I showered using regular soap with no perfumes or added scents. I preceded to get dressed in my looses pair of jeans, since I would be wearing those jeans the next day to go home if all went well. The looseness will accommodate the catheter and bag that I will leave the hospital with.

My son David took off from work to support my wife and I, which I thought was very cool.

Once loading everything in the car we would need for the over night stay. My wife and I secured the house and prepared to leave. I called my younger sister Tracye to tell her how to get there and the time of surgery.

It was raining so I decided to drive. Philadelphia traffic can be rough coming into the city especially if your not use to it. The drive was steady traffic of early morning commuters headed to Philadelphia.

I didn't get to see here before they took me back to the operating room prep area. I put on the hospital gown and the compression socks. They were warm and comfy.

As I lay there on the table talking away as they shaved my belly took my vitals and started an IV. I felt a little nervous but not to much. The people were very nice and smiled at some of my joking. Doctor Lee came in to say hi. Always good to see him. He always looked confident and happy, which I like from a doctor. I always call him the World Famous Doctor Lee and he just smiles. Not long after that I was getting sleepy, I believe I said goodbye to my wife who was sitting there watching everything, But the medication was kicking in. I don't even remember them putting the mask over my face to put me out.

I woke up three hours later in the recovery room. The first thing I heard a nurse say take deep breath David. I said to myself oh shit, you mean I'm not breathing. So I took a deep breath my eyes still closed. A few seconds later I heard her say it again. There was a machine near me beeping which stopped after I took a breath. Seconds later I hear the voice again, take a deep breath for me David. The breathing machine beeped again. Again I took a deep breath and the machine stopped. Eventually I just kept taking deep breaths until I was breathing on my own in a semi conscious state.

Not trying to scare you but during this type and probably many other operations where they don't want you to feel anything or have a reflex movement to pain your are very sedated to the point of not being able to control you own breathing. So the machine along with an anesthesiologist, controlled my breathing during the operation.

Next thing I remembered was waking up in my room. My wife was sitting in a chair next to me. My son was standing there and my sister. There wasn't much pain as I was lying there. I was still feeling the effects of the anesthesia from the operations five hours ago. I had a catheter installed in my penis up to my bladder for urination and a bag attached to it.

Nurses come every hour and check your vital signs blood pressure, heart rate, pain level. I was slow taking the meds because I wanted to feel how much pain I was in. That is until the pain started to raise my blood pressure, then the nurse and I thought it best that I take some. I never wanted to take to much because I wanted to feel some pain so I would know when I was doing to much moving around.

By 8:00 p.m. I wanted to get out of the bed. The nurse helped me to my feet. I had on special socks to prevent my blood from clotting, with an attachment that pressurized my legs and released like a pressure cuff does. That was disconnected when I took my walks

Once on my feet I felt I was on my way recovery. Walking was painful but tolerable. I was sore in my abdomen. Dragging the catheter around with the bag was a pain, one wrong move and it tugs and slides, ouch.

All I could think about was getting out of the hospital and home in my own bed. Which luckily for me if everything went well it would be the next day.

That night even with the drugs I couldn't sleep, which the nurses thought was odd. Most people blood pressure drops after surgery mine was high. I think that why I couldn't sleep. I don't like hospital beds either, because to me there not comfortable. I couldn't imagine being in one for a long time. Fortunately this operation is only requires a overnight stay unless there are complications that require you to stay longer.

During my stay I made a new friend named Jim, we walked the hallway together. I like to crack jokes although it was tearfully painful to laugh. However I forgot about that when I let one go.

Both Jim and I wrenched in pain when we attempted to laugh at my jokes. We couldn't even take a deep breath let along laugh. I tried to start a little competition with Jim on who could do the most laps around the floor. Jim alway won. I had to stop because of pain. Then I would tell Jim I need to lie down and rest. Jim would keep on walking.

That night my wife Kim got sick from some food she ate in a restaurant near the hospital. That worried me because she was suppose to drive me home tomorrow and it would have complicated me being able to leave. I stayed up almost all night playing with my phone taking pictures and posted one on Facebook of me in the hospital. I knew people would respond to that since I rarely get sick. Just trying to take my mind off my problems and the pains I was getting. I felt surrounded by angels the whole time I was there. The reason being, The building I was in or near was called the Wright Saunders building, which is my mothers married and maiden name. My nightshift nurse name was Kim, which is my wifes name. My dayshift nurse name was Valeria, which is my oldest sisters name. My doctors name is David, which is my name, and he is left handed like me. All coincidence, I don't think so. And rain has always been a blessing to me. It was raining the day I got married and I've been married for over thirty-five years.

CHAPTER 4

Check Out

Thursday morning check out day was here. I was happy, things were going as planned. I had to wait for Doctor Lee to see me before I could be released. My wife was feeling better as the day went on. I was happy about that. I was released around 4:00 p.m. and given prescriptions for pain. On my way out I thanked the nurses and stopped by Jim's room to wish him well. He told me he had to stick around a bit longer because he was in pain. All the extra walking and extra medicine masked some of the harm he was doing to himself. We exchanged numbers and I told him I would keep in touch.

The ride home was a bit painful because my pick up truck has a firm ride. Riding thru Philadelphia Center City is rough going around University Avenue. Especially after having prostate surgery. The catheter was getting on my nerves and I was cranky. Standing and sitting was a pain ful because the catheter slides.

My abdomen was practically unavailable to me due to the surgery. You don't realize how much you use those lovely muscles until you cant. Rolling in and out of bed took major effort. The first few days were painful and difficult. I was taking opioids the first week at home to deal with the variety of pains I was having. From my abs to my buttocks to urinating everything hurt. All that being said I haven't had a bowel movement in two days. How in the hell was I going to achieve that with abdominal pain and know abdominal strength. Stool softener thats how. The pain medicine works against you in this regard. They constipate you too.

I had trouble sleeping last night thinking about getting my catheter removed today. Even though I was 90 percent sure it would go well, its something you have to experience to truly appreciate. Still drinking more water than I ever have at any time of my life because it was important to flush my bladder. Outside it was raining and windy. I came downstairs to get a glass of water knowing I had to take my antibiotics today. The first pill had to be taken the morning of the

catheter removal, to prevent an infection from the catheter. I laid on the couch watching TV while I waited for 9:00 am to take the medicine. In the mean time I googled the drug to see what the side effects were. It didn't make me want to take it thats for sure. Levofloxacin was the antibiotic prescribed to be taken 1 per day in the morning same time each day for three days. The possible side effects are itching, facial swelling, rash, blistering, tingling in mouth or throat, nausea, vomiting, yellow skin or eyes, fainting, dizziness, severe headache, and seizures. So I sat there preparing myself for anything that might happen. 9:00 I took the oblong blue antibiotic pill and drank a full 16oz glass of water. Not long after I was curled up on the couch watching tv waiting for what ever effect I received. I noticed I was sleepy and slightly disoriented. Kim came down and asked if I wanted breakfast. I said ill take a a egg omlette with cheddar cheese and apple sauce. After eating I dosed off to sleep again right there on the couch. My appointment was at 2:00 pm in Philadelphia at the University of Pennsylvainia Medical Center. 11:00 I got off the couch to take a shower. After the shower I strapped a new portable bag to my leg and connected the catheter to the bag and got dressed. I didn't like the way the bag was feeling so I checked it. The bag was not filling with urine. I was puzzled because the hose was connected correctly. After checking it several times I realized there was a cap over the opening. Silly me how did I miss that I asked myself, was it the antibiotics, maybe I should have put my glasses on first. Small hurdles like that one mean a lot. I can only imagine what would have happened if I left the house with the bag like that.

Urine would have backed up in my bladder until I felt pressure or pain or both. Then I would have had to pull over on the highway to find out what was wrong, and probably get urine all over me in the process. At first I didn't want to drive but my wife wasn't feeling well so I decided to drive. She was getting a migraine headache. I could see the pain on her face. Suddenly it wasn't about me anymore I was worried about her instead. She had anti inflammatory pain reliever with her but no water. She managed to tough it out until we got to my appointment.

After we parked the car we made our way to the office appointment on the fourth floor and signed in at the kiosk station. I turned to see Jim and him wife standing in the waiting area. Jim told me he had already gotten his catheter removed and was standing there waiting to be able to urinate. Once you are able to pass urine you can leave. If you are unable to do so the catheter will have to be reinserted.. While talking to Jim and Kim about how things were going I got the call to go back to a room. I was ready to get it out. It was absolutely uncomfortable having it. When I'm nervous I tend to be quite chatty. Not sure why but it takes my mind off of me. A nurse assistant took all my vital signs and gave me a gown to put on. I laid back on the small bed and talked to my wife until Alice, Dr. Lee 'sassistant arrived. She came in and asked me a few general questions and perceeded to position me to remove the catheter. I knew already what she was going to do but didn't know how it would feel. The ballon which held the catheter in place would be deflated and a saline solution would be injected and catheter should come right out.

CHAPTER 5

Wiggle you toes

As she began to remove the catherter she told me to wiggle my toes. When I did she began to pulled the catheter out. That was the strangest feeling, the tube was longer that I realized. It felt like a long uncomfortable twinge. I said to Alice afterwards you told me to wiggle my toes to so I would be distracted didn't you. She nodded yes. Nice trick it worked I replied.

After that we talked a bit more about our families and stuff unrelated to my surgery. But Alice was busy and had more patients to see. She was easy to talk to and had a very pleasant personality.

She finished up by giving me further instructions an d my next appointments.

I went out to the lobby to wait for the moment I could pee. So I went to the water cooler to speed up the process. There was a black gentlemen sitting next to the cooler. We made eye contact and I spoke to him and gave him a fist bump. I could tell he was waiting for the same thing. He shook his head as if he wasn't sure if he did the right thing as far as getting the surgery. But I tried to assure him he did by saying now you'll probably out live everybody. About a minute after drinking the water I had to go. Everything came out ok, but it was stinging quite a bit, because my urethrea was sore from the catheter being in so long. I was glad on one had I could go. I was not happy with the burning sensation but I had the green light to go home.

CHAPTER 6

Incontinence

The next phase of the ordeal is incontinence. This phase put me in a diaper, oh my God, can this really be happening t me, It must be I told myself. Without the prostate, and the muscles associated with it to help you control urine flow, you will urinate very easily until you get your pelvic floor muscles under control and doing more work. They will be very weak from surgery and lack of use .There was a time before the operation I had to wait to go even when I had to go. Now its just the opposite, trying to stop going or continence is the problem now. Still better than a catheter by a mile. For me it took about a week and a half for the burning to stop when I urinated after the removal of the catheter.

I talked to Jim and he was having the same problem. Its invaluable to have a friend going thru the same thing. We can discuss each others progress and setbacks and support both.
I didn't like the diapers at all they fit and felt terrible. The mini pads aren't much better. For me its never where you need to be when you need it, even with the sticky on the back. I'm sure it works better for women because nothing is moving around like it is for a man.
Sometimes I'm awakened by the urge to pee, sometimes not. Thats annoying because I don't want to wear a pamper to bed. I'm a heavy sleeper so I need to feel the urge so I can get up in time.
Moreover standing or sitting down causes leaks to. Anything that causes pressure on the bladder can cause leakage. I've found that food moving past your bladder on its way to your colon will

apply pressure to the bladder also.

Certain foods will irritate the bladder giving you the urge to urinate when you don't have to. Drinks or food such as coffee, soda, citrus fruit and sugar can cause you to lose control of your bladder. The best thing to drink until you get incontinence under control is water. I had to give up anything with caffeine in it. Eventually I moved from diapers to heavy pads. I had to wear boxer briefs to support the pads where I normally would wear boxers. As time moved on progress was slow, but sure. I was able to stop using pads all the time. Definitely a cause for celebration. But I found that each day could be different. Depending on how much sleep you get, how tired you are, the food you ate etc. Dr. Lee told me it would take a year to fully heal, and he was right. I'm coming up on 10 months and I still leak a little. But it is slowing and getting better every month. Today as I write this chapter I feel the best control Ive felt since before surgery.

CHAPTER 7

Follow Up

After surgery while your home healing and trying to adjust to the new me. There comes a time when you have to be blood tested again to make sure the cancer is gone. This was a nervous time for me because I had to prepare for bad news if there was going to be any. Although everyone I spoke with, that had been through the surgery, assured me that my results would be negative. And they were right. I was confident that the results would be okay because according to the scans that were done the cancer was limited to the prostate as far as that test could tell. But there is always a chance they missed something. I had blood work done 3 months after surgery and a appointment to see Dr. Lee to discuss the test results and answer any questions I might have. The test results score was 0.06. A perfect score, I was my old self again, relieved and very happy. I didn't really have any questions, I was all smiles at the results and congratulated Dr. Lee. I filled out a questionnaire that asked me an important question. The question was, if I had to live with my current situation would I be ok with it. Meaning the leakage I was experiencing today, could I live with it. I answered yes but I wasn't being sincere. I just didn't want any more treatments of any kind. And I hoped that he wasn't implying that I wasn't going to get any better than my current situation. The good news was there was no cancer present in my blood. I felt very relieved to say the least. Cause for celebration for sure. Time went on and I continued to struggle with incontenence. I was getting so tired of it. I started to believe it will be something ill just have to live with. Ive had my low moments in my life but I always found away to rise above them.

Three more months went by and again I go in for blood work, actually I was almost two months late getting the blood work done. I guess I was prepared for any bad news. I should have got it done in late August but didn't move on it until November. Fortunately I didn't have to go to Philadelphia for a face to face. Only had to go to lab corp and they will forward the labs to the doctor and they will send me the results thru there portal which I am a member of. Hoorah the results were 0.06 again, beautiful.

CHAPTER 8

Clothes Dryer

My grandson Marcus is sick with some type of stomach virus. My daughter, his mother is nursing a precious new born name Zariyah, his little sister. 'She came over with them, after the doctors appointment. She left him in the car. Even though I didn't want any company until I felt better I told her to bring him in the house I want to take a look at him. I knew it would be hard to take care of him with a nursing baby in her arms. He was really sick. He couldn't keep anything down, he couldn't drink or eat anything. I set up the back room for him to sleep in as we tried to figure out what to give him. My wife who loves him dearly took over some of the nursing care of him along with my daughter. However he was getting any better as far as I could tell. At times contemplated taking him back to the hospital. To see him in such misery was alarming for me. I went to the drug store to get a prescription filled for upset stomach and vomiting.

In the mean time I could heard my gas clothes dryer making a strange noise, and everyone else heard it to. My daughter Alesia asked me what was that noise. I sadly said its the dryer, So I went downstairs to the basement to check on it. It was shutting off without finishing the clothes drying. Great, first the air conditioner, then the hot water heater, now this. I was getting upset about all that was happening now that I'm incapacitated. Luckily I was able to fix the air conditioner myself. There were wires cut from my grandson Jaymier using the weed wacker to close to to the wiring.

I know I have to be careful what I do as far as work until I heal up completely, but these things need imediate attention or quality of life suffers..

I have fixed this dryer before when the burner failed and when the belt broke. I new the inner working pretty good I thought. I talked to my friend Dwayne about it and he told me don't do it because I might injure myself. I told him I felt good enough to to do it. I took his advice and called a service man out for 100.00 dollars to give me a estimate for repairs.

He told me the motor was bad and, in order to guarantee the work I had to replace other parts to.

Like the fan attached to the motor and the drum pulleys for a total of 385.00 dollars. Dude I can by a new dryer for that kind of money. He agreed with me. I paid him for his estimate and sent him on his way. One thing I got from his visit is to get some paper booties he wore on his boots for working in the house.

I decided to get a price for the motor, it was 100.00 dollars. I figure ill save some money and put it in myself. 200.00 investment so far. The motor was a pain to get out of the dryer because of the plastic blower motor attached to the motor shaft. The nut actually stripped because the blower was on so tight. So I had to order a new one. 29.00 dollars. The blower came and I had to chisel the old one off the motor shaft to put the new one on. Of course I'm lying on the ground and twisting and pulling. I managed to get the motor in and the fan on to. Unfortunately after putting the dryer back together it ran fine except now it wont light. I wanted to scream. It was lighting before. What did I do wrong to cause it not to want to light anymore. Im thinking this is to much. I should have just brought a new dryer and called it a day.

In the days that follow sore again internally. No blood but I feel pain like I shouldn't have done it. Almost to the point of pain medicine.

Since the dryer was half part I decided after talking to a rep on the phone that ignitor is a fragile piece and it make have gotten damaged while I was disasembling the dryer. So I took a chance and order it after testing the ignitor for proper resistance. The reading was close to normal. The ignitor was there in a days time. I installed it and tried to run the dryer. The dryer spun fine but still wouldnt lite the burner. Then I found a wire off its connection in the back of the dryer. I look all over the back of the dryer to find where it had come off with no success. The decision was made by myself to replace the dryer and return the parts.

CHAPTER 9

Long Distance Friend

There is a person representing groups of people seven hundred miles away who are interested in my progress. This person is the company nurse from my companies medical department. Although it appeared she generally cared about my progress, there is a underlying agenda. That hidden agenda was getting me back to work before long term disability kicks in. It was her job to make sure that it didnt occur. Her method was to get my doctor to release me even if I wasn't completely ready to go back to work, under the guise of some sort of light duty workstatus of which my employer doesn't have. Even though my doctor had given me a release date of eight weeks, they were pressing for six week return. This conversation was happening three weeks after surgery which made me fighting mad since I was still in pain and discomfort every part of my day and night. She even threatened to stop my benefits if my doctor did not comply with her demands.

I called my Operations Manager to ask what is the problem with this company nurse and he big push for me to return to work before I was ready. He was just as surprised as I so it seemed. And after telling him, I'm about to write her a nasty gram and he told me to copy him on it, which I did. He also said that he didn't expect me back until October and that they were fine. So apparently the pressure was not coming from him or my department heads. I just wanted to confirm that before I went in on a nurse five hundred miles away. In there defense I'm sure there are those who try to abuse there disability benefits. But that is not my character, and i take offense to the implication. I'm sure there are those who are on disability with little or no need for it. Thats no excuse for harassing me and treating me like a criminal.

CHAPTER 10

Ready for work

The time has come to return to work, its been eight weeks and it's showtime. Incontinence is the most difficult problem now. If I can overcome this I will be golden. I haven't been practicing my Kegel exercises like I should. I keep forgetting to do them. But I will have to try harder. Of course, like everything else along this path takes time and patience to. You can't really rush it. If you could I would have done it.

Everyone is supportive of the process I'm going through. My body does feel different. My body likes food more than before. I attribute that to the fact that its still healing from surgery and wants the nutrition that the food provides to accomplish it. Fact is if I go too long without eating I will get tired more quickly and feel sickly if I don't do something about it. I think this will go away once my body completely heals, but we will see.

I still haven't tried to lift anything heavy but I think I will try some free weights after a little moor time, just to see how my body, muscles and bladder respond.

I was taking the drug Cialis as prescribed buy Dr. Lee. but stopped because I though I didn't need it because I was getting erections without it. However after speaking to Dr. Lee I resumed taking it. He has the expertise on these matters and I trust what he says. He informed me that men who use the drug during the first year, recover much better than those who don't use it. It is quite expensive though $125 dollars for a 60 day supply even with insurance. It's suppose increases blood flow to the areas involved in surgery thereby allowing better and faster healing. I don't feel any different after taking it but what do I know. Work is a struggle because of incontinence. It seems that I am able to control it until the muscles get tired. Normally about halfway through the day. So rest has become even more important. In my case rest is more difficult to get because I work 12 hour shifts with overtime. For guys with a regular work week in should be a bit easier to handle. Certain foods that if avoided will help bladder control. Like citrus fruits, caffeine, and sugar. These will cause bladder irritation which will give you the feeling of needing to urinate when you don't. There are a number of absorbent pads on the market that you will need until you heal more and the Kegel muscles get stronger and control more. I always keep some with me. There hit or miss, because the penis is not always in position to make use of the pad in my experience. The work situation is a personal one because no one knows why you were out of work unless you tell them. I thought everyone knew why I as out but they didn't seem to know. I did talk about it. Its hard for me not to. It was a life changing experience and I wanted to let other men know to get checked and why.

CHAPTER 11

Erectile Function

Okay lets talk about erections. This of course is a area of great importance to me or any man. However under the circumstances it wasn't the primary concern as one might expect. Mostly because if you can't control urination, Intimacy with your significant other is not so desirable a situation, if at all possible. The human body is an amazing. In this department one function is cut off when the other function starts. In other words you can't urinate with and erection. The body shuts down urination while you have and erection. So once you can control urination you can ease on into intimacy with more confidence.

For me that was one of the biggest hurdles. The exercises are a pain to do but are very important to strengthening the Kegel muscle.

My doctors encouraged me to engage in sex. Ive heard of cases where sex is not recommended for some time after surgery. In my case according to my doctors I should try.

I have been able to achieve erections, not as firm as before but there are other factors in that equation. Such as high blood pressure medicines (beta blockers) like lisinopril which was prescribed by my primary physican for high blood pressure.

Cialis was prescribed by my surgeon to assist in the healing of my surgery and the nerves associated with the quality of my erections. Even though I was able to achieve and good erection I took my doctors advice. Last week I went for a annual health screening examination given by my employer, there was some hearing loss identified in my left ear. Which was different from my last years hearing test. Prior to my surgery. I was thinking because I had a cold and some congestion in my sinuses it could be the reason for the low hearing score in my left ear. Even so I started to pay more attention to my ears. There was and occasional ringing in my ear along with a hissing sound much like you hear in a seashell. As much as I hate to read the side effects of drugs I had to take a look at the side effects of Cialis. Turns out that sudden or gradual hearing loss is possible when taking the drug. I had my hearing checked by a ENT doctor and asked him if it is possible and he told me yes it can cause it.

I stopped taking it and my ear ringing cleared up and, I still get good erections. However I have made changes to my diet also. I am not a vegetarian but I definitely eat less meat products, and more vegetables and grains instead. Exercise is also important to your cardio vascular health which directly affects erectile functions.

CHAPTER 12

One Year

One year later I'm still dealing with the changes to my body but managing well. I realize the instructions that were given to me were correct, especially about the foods to avoid. If you go through the process I'm sure you will agree. Caffeine is not your friend anymore. I love coffee, but I'm avoiding it, at least for now because it makes me go almost without warning, along with sugar and chocolate which has caffeine as well.

There were plenty of questions asked by my doctor on a questionnaire. When you go in for your one year follow up appointment. For example, if you had to deal with the level of leakage you're presently experiencing, for the rest of your life, would you be allright with it? I answered that question yes. My philosophy to adversity is to align myself mentally with the situations to grow from the experience, to build physical and mental strength. Instead of pity and self doubt. Bring a positive attitude and a positive outlook. That philosophy turns adversity into opportunity.

However I think what amazes me the most, is the amount of time it takes for the body to recover from major surgery.

It takes years to get your body back to the level of strength that you were use to, especially the abdomen. Fact is even exercise which is essential for the health of body is limited by the healing process.

It takes about two years for your body to completely heal after this type of surgery. Another obstacle during the healing process is weight gain. I contributed the additional weight gain to of course my increased eating and limited exercise.

The healing requires you to eat, I would start to get sick if I missed meals or tried intermittent fasting. Which I would do often before I had the surgery. So the balance between eating, resting, and sleeping changed while I was healing. You can almost measure the healing by how I feel without food during periods of intermittent fasting.

In closing I will say, if you have been diagnosed with prostate cancer and are considering the prostectiomy option. You will be in good company. I know plenty of men living productive sexually active lives after the surgery myself included. And if you happen to reading this book and you have not been tested for prostate cancer. Make plans to get tested, the earlier the better so it doesnt have a chance to spread to other parts of the body.

www.ingramcontent.com/pod-product-compliance
Lightning Source LLC
Chambersburg PA
CBHW030555220526
45463CB00007B/3084